FROM PASSION TO PEACE

James Allen

HAWK PRESS

Published by

Hawk Press
4836/24, Ansari Road, Daryaganj
New Delhi – 110 002
Phones: +91-11-23278618, +91-11-43667199
E-mail: thehawkpress@gmail.com
www.thehawkpress.com

ISBN: 978-93-88841-39-9

CONTENTS

Foreword

THE first three parts of this book, Passion, Aspiration, and Temptation, represent the common human life, with its passion, pathos, and tragedy; the last three parts, Transcendence, Beatitude, and Peace, present the Divine Life — calm, wise, and beautiful — of the sage and Saviour. The middle part, Transmutation, is the transitional stage between the two; it is the alchemic process linking the divine with the human life. Discipline, denial, and renunciation do not constitute the Divine State; they are only the means by which it is attained. The Divine Life is established in that Perfect Knowledge which bestows Perfect Peace.

James Allen
Bryngoleu
Ilfracombe, Devon.
England

PASSION

The pathway of the saints and sages; the road of the wise and pure; the highway along which the Saviours have trod, and which all Saviours to come will also walk — such is the subject of this book; such is the high and holy theme which the author briefly expounds in these pages.

Passion is the lowest level of human life. None can descend lower. In its chilling swamps and concealing darkness creep and crawl the creatures of its sunless world. Lust, hatred, covetousness, pride, vanity, greed, revenge, envy, spite, retaliation, slander, backbiting, lying, theft, deceit, treachery, cruelty, suspicion, jealousy — such are the brute forces and blind, unreasoning impulses that inhabit the underworld of passion, and roam, devouring and devoured, in the rank primeval jungles of the human mind.

There also dwell the dark shapes of remorse and pain and suffering, and the drooping forms of grief and sorrow and lamentation.

In this dark world the unwise live and die, not knowing the peace of purity, nor the joy of that Divine Light which forever shines above them, and for them, yet shines in vain so long as it falls on unseeing eyes which look not up, but are ever bent earthward — flesh ward.

But the wise look up. They are not satisfied with this passion-world, and they bend their steps towards the upper world of peace, the light and glory of which they behold, at first afar off, but nearer and with ever increasing splendor as they ascend.

None can fall lower than passion, but all can rise higher. In that lowest place where further descent is impossible, all who move forward must ascend; and the ascending pathway is always at hand, near, and easily accessible. It is the way of self-conquest, and he has already entered it who has begun to say "nay" to his selfishness, who has begun to discipline his desires, and to control and command the unruly elements of his mind.

Passion is the arch-enemy of mankind, the slayer of happiness, the opposite and enemy of peace. From it proceeds all that defiles and destroys. It is the source of suffering, the maker of misery, and the promulgator of mischief and disaster.

The inner world of selfishness is rooted in ignorance, — ignorance of Divine Law, of Divine Goodness; ignorance of the Pure Way and the Peaceful Path. Passion is dark, and it thrives and flourishes in spiritual darkness. It cannot enter the regions of spiritual light. In the enlightened mind the darkness of ignorance is destroyed; in the pure heart there is no place for passion.

Passion in all its forms is a mental thirst, a fever, a torturing unrest. As a fire consumes a magnificent building, reducing it to a heap of unsightly ashes, so are men consumed by the flames of passions, and their deeds and works fall and perish.

If one would find peace, he must come out of passion. The wise man subdues his passions, the foolish man is subdued by them. The seeker for wisdom begins by turning his back on folly. The lover of peace enters the way which leads thereto, and with every step he takes he leaves further below and behind him the dark dwelling-place of passion and despair.

The first step towards the heights of wisdom and peace is to understand the darkness and misery of selfishness, and when that is understood, the overcoming it — the coming out of it — will follow.

Selfishness, or passion, not only subsists in the gross forms of greed and glaringly ungoverned conditions of mind; it informs also every hidden thought which is subtly connected with the assumption and glorification of one's self; and it is most deceiving and subtle when it prompts one to dwell upon the selfishness in others, to accuse them of it and to talk about it. The man who continually dwells upon the selfishness in others will not thus overcome his own selfishness. Not by accusing others do we come out of selfishness, but by purifying ourselves. The way from passion to peace is not by hurling painful charges against others, but by overcoming one's self. By eagerly striving to subdue the selfishness of others, we remain passion-bound; by patiently overcoming our own selfishness, we ascend into freedom. He only who has conquered himself can subdue others; and he subdues them, not by passion, but by love. The foolish man accuses others and justifies himself; but he who is becoming wise justifies others and accuses himself. The way from passion to peace is not in the outer world of people; it is in the inner world of thoughts; it does not consist in altering the deeds of others, it consists in perfecting one's own deeds.

Frequently the man of passion is most eager to put others right; but the man of wisdom puts himself right. If one is anxious to reform the world, let him begin by reforming himself The reformation of self does not end with the elimination of the sensual elements only; that is its beginning. It ends only when every vain thought and selfish aim is overcome. Short of perfect:

purity and wisdom, there is still some form of self-slavery or folly which needs to be conquered.

Passion is at the base of the structure of life; peace is its crown and summit. Without passion to begin with, there would be no power to work with, and no achievement to end with. Passion represents power, but power misdirected, power producing hurt instead of happiness. Its forces, while being instruments of destruction in the hands of the foolish, are instruments of preservation in the hands of the wise. When curbed and concentrated and beneficently directed, they represent working energy. Passion is the flaming sword which guards the gates of Paradise. It shuts out and destroys the foolish; it admits and preserves the wise.

He is the foolish man who does not know the extent of his own ignorance; who is the slave of thoughts of self; who obeys the impulses of passion. He is the wise man who knows his own ignorance; who understands the emptiness of selfish thoughts; who masters the impulses of passion.

The fool descends into deeper and deeper ignorance; the wise man ascends into higher and higher knowledge. The fool desires, and suffers, and dies. The wise man aspires, and rejoices, and lives.

With mind intent on wisdom, and mental gaze raised upward, the spiritual warrior perceives the upward way, and fixes his attention upon the heights of Peace.

ASPIRATION

With the clear perception of one's own ignorance, comes the desire for enlightenment, and thus in the heart is born Aspiration, the rapture of the saints.

On the wings of aspiration man rises from earth to heaven, from ignorance to knowledge, from the under darkness to the upper light. Without it he remains a grovelling animal, earthly, sensual, unenlightened, and uninspired.

Aspiration is the longing for heavenly things — for righteousness, compassion, purity, love — as distinguished from desire, which is the longing for earthly things, — for selfish possessions, personal dominance, low pleasures, and sensual gratifications.

As a bird deprived of its wings cannot soar, so a man without aspiration cannot rise above his surroundings and become master of his animal inclinations. He is the slave of passions, is subject to others, and is carried hither and thither by the changing current of events.

For one to begin to aspire means that he is dissatisfied with his low estate, and is aiming at a higher condition. It is a sure sign that he is roused out of his lethargic sleep of animality, and has become conscious of nobler attainments and a fuller life.

Aspiration makes all things possible. It opens the way to advancement. Even the highest state of perfection conceivable it brings near and makes real and possible; for that which can be conceived can be achieved.

Aspiration is the twin angel to inspiration. It unlocks the gates of joy. Singing accompanies soaring. Music, poetry, prophecy, and all high and holy instruments, are at last placed in the hands of him whose aspirations flag not, whose spirit does not fail.

So long as animal conditions taste sweet to a man, he cannot aspire; he is so far satisfied; but when their sweetness turns to bitterness, then in his sorrow he thinks of nobler things. When he is deprived of earthly joy, he aspires to the joy which is heavenly. It is when impurity turns to suffering that purity is sought. Truly aspiration rises, phoenix-like, from the dead ashes of repentance, but on its powerful pinions man can reach the heaven of heavens.

The man of aspiration has entered the way which ends in peace; and surely he will reach that end if he stays not nor turns back. If he constantly renews his mind with glimpses of the heavenly vision, he will reach the heavenly state.

Man attains in the measure that he aspires. His longing to be is the gauge of what he can be. To Fix the mind is to foreordain the achievement. As man can experience and know all low things, so he can experience and know all high things. As he has become human, so he can become divine. The turning of the mind in high and divine directions is the sole and needful task.

What is impurity but the impure thoughts of the thinker? What is purity but the pure thoughts of the thinker? One man does not do the thinking of another. Each man is pure or impure of himself alone.

If a man thinks, "It is through others, or circumstances, or heredity that I am impure," how can he hope to overcome his errors? Such a thought will check all holy aspirations, and bind him to the slavery of passion.

When a man fully perceives that his errors and impurities are his own, that they are generated and fostered by himself, that he alone is responsible for them, then he will aspire to overcome them, the way of attainment will be opened up to him, and he will see whence and whither he is travelling.

The man of passion sees no straight path before him, and behind him all is fog and gloom. He seizes the pleasure of the moment, and does not strive for understanding or think of wisdom. His way is confused, turbulent, troubled, and his heart is far from peace.

The man of aspiration sees before him the pathway up the heavenly heights, and behind him are the circuitous routes of passion up which he has hitherto blindly groped. Striving for understanding, and his mind set on wisdom, his way is clear, and his heart already experiences a foretaste of the final peace.

Men of passion strive mightily to achieve little things, — things which speedily perish, and, in the place where they were, leave nothing to be remembered.

Men of aspiration strive with equal might to achieve great things — things of virtue, of knowledge, of wisdom, which do not perish, but stand as monuments of inspiration for the uplifting of mankind.

As the merchant achieves worldly success by persistent exertion, so the saint achieves spiritual success by aspiration and endeavor. One becomes a merchant, the other a saint, by the particular direction in which his mental energy is guided.

When the rapture of aspiration touches the mind, it at once refines it, and the dross of its impurities begins to fall away; yea, while aspiration holds the mind, no impurity can enter it, for the impure and the pure cannot at the same moment occupy the thought. But the effort of aspiration is at first spasmodic and short-lived. The mind falls back into its habitual error, and must be constantly renewed.

The lover of the pure life renews his mind daily with the invigorating glow of aspiration. He rises early, and fortifies his mind with strong thoughts and strenuous endeavor. He knows that the mind is of such a nature that it cannot remain for a moment unoccupied, and that if it is not held and guided by high thoughts and pure aspirations, it will assuredly be enslaved and misguided by low thoughts and base desires.

Aspiration can be fed, fostered, and strengthened by daily habit, just as is desire. It can be sought, and admitted into the mind as a divine guide, or it can be neglected and shut out. To retire for a short time each day to some quiet spot, preferably in the open air, and there call up the energies of the mind in surging waves of holy rapture, is to prepare the mind for great spiritual victories and destinies of divine import; for such rapture is the preparation for wisdom and the prelude to peace. Before the mind can contemplate pure things it must be lifted up to them, it must rise above impure things ; and aspiration is the instrument by which this is accomplished. By its aid the mind soars swiftly and surely into heavenly places, and begins to experience divine things; begins to accumulate wisdom, and to learn to guide itself by an ever increasing measure of the divine light of pure knowledge.

To thirst for righteousness; to hunger for the pure life; to rise in holy rapture on the wings of angelic aspiration — this is the right road to wisdom; this is the right striving for peace; this is the right beginning of the way divine.

TEMPTATION

Aspiration can carry a man into heaven, but to remain there he must learn to conform his entire mind to the heavenly conditions: to this end temptation works.

Temptation is the reversion, in thought, from purity to passion. It is a going back from aspiration to desire. It threatens aspiration until the point is reached where desire is quenched in the waters of pure knowledge and calm thought. In the early stages of aspiration, temptation is subtle and powerful, and is regarded as an enemy ; but it is only an enemy in the sense that the tempted one is his own enemy. In the sense that it is the revealer of weakness and impurity, it is a friend, a necessary factor in spiritual training. It is, indeed, an accompaniment of the effort to overcome evil and apprehend good. To be successfully conquered, the evil in a man must come to the surface and present itself, and it is in temptation that the evil hidden in the heart stands revealed and exposed.

That which temptation appeals to and arouses is unconquered desire, and temptation will again and again assail and subdue a man until he has lifted himself above the lusting impulses. Temptation is an appeal to the impure. That which is pure cannot be subject to temptation.

Temptation waylays the man of aspiration until he touches the region of the divine consciousness, and beyond that border temptation cannot follow him. It is when a man begins to aspire that he begins to be tempted. Aspiration rouses up all the latent good and evil, in order that the man may be fully revealed to himself, for a man cannot overcome himself unless he fully knows himself It can scarcely be said of the merely animal man that he is tempted, for the very presence of temptation means that there is a striving for a purer state. Animal desire and gratification is the normal condition of the man who has not yet risen into aspiration; he wishes for nothing more, nothing better, than his sensual enjoyments, and is, for the present, satisfied. Such a man cannot be tempted to fall, for he has not yet risen.

The presence of aspiration signifies that a man has taken one step, at least, upward, and is therefore capable of being drawn back, and this backward attraction is called temptation. The allurements of temptation subsist in the impure thoughts and downward desires of the heart. The object of temptation is powerless to attract when the heart no longer lusts for it. The stronghold of temptation is within a man, not without; and until a man realizes this, the period of temptation will be protracted. While a man continues to run away from outward objects, under the delusion that temptation subsists entirely in them, and does not attack and purge away his impure imaginings, his temptations will increase, and his falls will be many and grievous. When a man clearly perceives that the evil is within, and not without, then his progress will be rapid, his temptations will decrease, and the final overcoming of all temptation will be well within the range of his spiritual vision.

Temptation is torment. It is not an abiding condition, but is a passage from a lower condition to a higher. The fulness and perfection of life is bliss, not torment. Temptation accompanies weakness and defeat, but a man is destined for strength and victory. The presence of torment is the signal to rise and conquer. The man of persistent and ever renewed aspiration does not allow himself to think that temptation cannot be overcome. He is determined to be master of himself Resignation to evil is an acknowledgment of defeat. It signifies that the battle against self is abandoned; that good is denied; that evil is made supreme.

As the energetic man of business is not daunted by difficulties, but studies how to overcome them, so the man of ceaseless aspiration is not crushed into submission by temptations, but meditates how he may fortify his mind; for the tempter is like a coward, he only creeps in at weak and unguarded points.

The tempted one should study thoughtfully the nature and meaning of temptation, for until it is known it cannot be overcome. A wise general, before attacking the opposing force, studies the tactics of his enemy; so he who is to overcome temptation must understand how it arises in his own darkness and error, and must study, by introspection and meditation, how to disperse the darkness and supplant error by truth.

The stronger a man's passions, the fiercer will be his temptations ; the deeper his selfishness, the more subtle his temptations; the more pronounced his vanity, the more flattering and deceptive his temptations.

A man must know himself if he is to know truth. He must not shrink from any revelation which will expose his error; on the contrary, he must welcome such revelations as aids to that self-knowledge which is the handmaid of self-conquest.

The man who cannot endure to have his errors and shortcomings brought to the surface and made known, but tries to hide them, is unfit to walk the highway of truth. He is not properly equipped to battle with and overcome temptation. He who cannot fearlessly face his lower nature cannot climb the rugged heights of renunciation.

Let the tempted one know this: that he himself is both tempter and tempted; that all his enemies are within; that the flatterers which seduce, the taunts which stab, and the flames which burn, all spring from that inner region of ignorance and error in which he has hitherto lived; and knowing this, let him be assured of complete victory over evil. When he is sorely tempted, let him not mourn, therefore, but let him rejoice in that his strength is tried and his weakness exposed. For he who truly knows and humbly acknowledges his weakness will not be slow in setting about the acquisition of strength.

Foolish men blame others for their lapses and sins, but let the truth-lover blame only himself. Let him acknowledge his complete responsibility for his own conduct, and not say, when he falls, this thing, or such and such circumstance, or that man, was to blame; for the most which others can do is to afford an opportunity for our own good or evil to manifest itself; they cannot make us good or evil.

Temptation is at first sore, grievous, and hard to be borne, and subtle and persistent is the assailant; but if the tempted one is firm and courageous, and does not give way, he will gradually subdue his spiritual enemy, and will finally triumph in the knowledge of good.

The adverse one is compounded of a man's own lust and selfishness and pride, and when these are put away, evil is seen to be as naught, and good is revealed in all-victorious splendor.

TRANSMUTATION

Midway between the hell of Passion and the heaven of Peace is the purgatory of Transmutation, — not a speculative purgatory beyond the grave, but a real purgatory in the human heart. In its separating and purifying fire the base metal of error is sifted away, and only the clarified gold of truth remains.

When temptation has culminated in sorrow and deep perplexity, then the tempted one, strenuously striving for deliverance, finds that his thraldom is entirely from himself, and that instead of fighting against outer circumstances, he must alter inner conditions. The fight against outer things is necessary at the commencement. It is the only course which can be adopted at the first, because of the prevailing ignorance of mental causation, but it never, of itself, brings about emancipation. What it does bring about is the knowledge of the mental cause of temptation ; and the knowledge of the mental cause of temptation leads to the transmutation of thought, and the transmutation of thought leads to deliverance from the bondage of error.

The preliminary fighting is a necessary stage in spiritual development, as the crying and kicking of a helpless babe is necessary to its growth; but as the crying and kicking is not needed beyond the infant stage, so the fierce struggling with, and falling under, temptation ends when the knowledge of mental transmutation is acquired.

The truly wise man, he who is enlightened concerning the source and cause of temptation, does not fight against outward allurements, he abandons all desire for them; they thus cease to be allurements, and the power of temptation is destroyed at its source. But this abandonment of unholy desire is not a final process, it is the beginning of a regenerative and transforming power which, patiently employed, leads man to the clear and cloudless heights of spiritual enlightenment.

Spiritual transmutation consists in an entire reversal of the ordinary self-seeking attitude of mind towards men and things, and this reversal brings about an entirely new set of experiences. Thus the desire for a certain pleasure is abandoned, cut off at its source, and not allowed to have any place in the consciousness; but the mental force which that desire represented is not annihilated, it is transferred to a higher region of thought, transmuted into a purer form of energy. The law of conservation of energy obtains universally in mind as in matter, and the force shut off in lower directions is liberated in higher realms of spiritual activity.

Along the Saintly Way towards the divine life, the midway region of Transmutation is the Country of Sacrifice, it is the Plain of Renunciation. Old passions, old desires, old ambitions and thoughts, are cast away and abandoned, but only to reappear in some more beautiful, more permanent, more eternally satisfying form. As valuable jewels, long guarded and cherished, are thrown tearfully into the melting-pot, yet are remoulded into new and more perfect adornments, so the spiritual alchemist, at first loth to part company with long-cherished thoughts and habits, at last gives them up, to discover, a little later, to his joy, that they have come back to him in the form of new faculties, rarer powers, and purer joys, — spiritual jewels newly burnished, beautiful and resplendent.

In transmuting his mind from evil to good, a man comes to distinguish more and more clearly between error and Truth, and so distinguishing, he ceases to be swayed and prompted by outward things, and by the actions and attitudes of others; he acts from his knowledge of truth. First acknowledging his errors, and then confronting them with a searching mind and a humble heart, he subdues, conquers, and transmutes them.

The early stage of transmutation is painful but brief, for the pain is soon transformed into pure spiritual joy, the brevity of the pain being measured by the intelligence and energy with which the process is pursued.

While a man thinks that the cause of his pain is in the attitude of others, he will not pass beyond it, but when he perceives that its cause is in himself, then he will pass beyond it into joy.

The unenlightened man allows himself to be disturbed, wounded, and overthrown by what he regards as the wrong attitude of others towards him ; this is because the same wrong attitude is in himself. He, indeed, metes out to them, in return, the same actions, regarding as right in himself that which is wrong in others. Slander is given for slander, hatred for hatred, anger for anger. This is the action and reaction of evil; it is the clash of selfishness with selfishness. It is only the self, or selfish elements, within a man that can be aroused by the evil in another; the Truth, or divine characteristics, in a man cannot be approached by that evil, much less can it be disturbed and overthrown by it.

It is the conversion, or complete reversal, of this self into Truth that constitutes Transmutation. The enlightened man has abandoned the delusion that the evil in others has power to hurt and subdue him, and he has grasped the profound truth that he is only overthrown by the evil in himself He therefore ceases to blame others for his sins and sufferings, and applies himself to purifying his own heart. In this reversal of his mental attitude, he transmutes the lower selfish forces into the higher moral attributes. The base ore of error is cast into the fire of sacrifice, and there comes forth the pure gold of Truth.

Such a man stands firm and unmoved when assailed by outward things. He is self's master, not its slave. He has ceased to identify himself with the impulses of passion, and has identified himself with Truth. He has overcome evil, and has become merged in Good. He knows both error and Truth, and has abandoned error and brought himself into harmony with Truth. He returns good for evil. The more he is assailed by evil from without, the greater is his opportunity of manifesting the good from within. That which supremely differentiates the fool from the wise man is this, — that the fool meets passion with passion, hatred with hatred, and returns evil for evil; whereas the wise man meets passion with peace, hatred with love, and returns good for evil.

Men inflict sufferings upon themselves through the active instrumentality of their own unpurified nature. They rise into perfect peace in the measure that they purify their hearts. The mental energy which men waste in the pursuance of dark passions is all-sufficient to enable them to reach the highest wisdom when it is turned in the right direction. As water, when transmuted into steam, becomes a new, more definite and wide-reaching power, so passion, when transmuted into intellectual and moral force, becomes a new life, a new power for the accomplishment of high and unfailing purposes.

Mental forces, like molecular, have their opposite poles or modes of action, and where the negative pole is, there also is the positive. Where ignorance is, wisdom is possible; where passion abounds, peace awaits ; where there is much suffering, much bliss is near. Sorrow is the negation of joy; sin is the opposite of purity; evil is the denial of good. Where there is an opposite, there is that which is opposed. The adverse evil, in its denial of the good, testifies to its presence. The one thing needful, therefore, is the turning round from the negative to the positive ; the conversion of the heart from impure desires to pure aspirations; the transmutation of the passional forces into moral powers.

The wise purify their thoughts; they turn from bad deeds, and do good deeds; they put error behind them, and approach Truth. Thus do they rise above the allurements of sin, above the torments of temptation, above the dark world of sorrow, and enter the Divine Consciousness, the Transcendent Life.

TRANSCENDENCE

When a man passes from the dark stage of temptation to the more enlightened stage of transmutation, he has become a saint; namely, one who perceives the need of self-purification, who understands the way of self-purification, and who has entered that way and is engaged in perfecting himself. But there comes a time in the process of transmutation when, with the decrease of evil and the accumulation of good, there dawns in the mind a new vision, a new consciousness, a new man. And when this is reached, the saint has become a sage; he has passed from the human life to the divine life. He is "born again," and there begins for him a new round of experiences; he wields a new power; a new universe opens out before his spiritual gaze. This is the stage of Transcendence ; this I call the Transcendent Life.

When there is no more consciousness of sin; when anxiety and doubt, and grief and sorrow, are ended; when lust and enmity, and anger and envy, no more possess the thoughts; when there remains in the mind no vestige of blame towards others for one's own condition, and when all conditions are seen to be good because the result of causes, so that no event can afflict the mind, then Transcendence is attained ; then the limited human personality is outgrown, and the divine life is known; evil is transcended, and Good is all-in-all.

The divine consciousness is not an intensification of the

human, it is a new form of consciousness. It springs from the old, but it is not a continuance of it. Born of the lower life of sin and sorrow, after a period of painful travail, it yet transcends that life, and has no part in it, as the perfect flower transcends the seed from which it sprang.

As passion is the keynote of the self-life, so serenity is the keynote of the transcendent life. Rising into it, man is lifted above inharmony and disturbance. When Perfect Good is realized and known, not as an opinion or an idea, but as an experience, a possession, then calm vision is acquired, and tranquil joy abides through all vicissitudes. The transcendent life is ruled, not by passions, but by principles. It is founded, not upon fleeting impulses, but upon abiding laws. In its clear atmosphere, the orderly sequence of all things is revealed, so that there is seen to be no room for sorrow, anxiety, or regret. While men are involved in the passions of self, they load themselves with cares, and trouble over many things; and more than all else do they trouble over their own little, burdened, pain-stricken personality, being anxious for its fleeting pleasures, for its protection and preservation, and for its eternal safety and continuance. Now in the life that is wise and good all this is transcended. Personal interests are replaced by universal purposes, and all cares, troubles, and anxieties concerning the pleasure and fate of the personality are dispelled like the feverish dreams of a night.

Passion is blind and ignorant; it sees and knows only its own gratification. Self recognizes no law; its object is to get and to enjoy. The getting is a graduated scale varying from sensual greed, through many subtle vanities, up to the desire for a personal heaven or personal immortality, but it is self still; it is the old sensual craving coming out again in a more subtle and deceptive form; it is the longing for some personal delight, along with its accompanying dread lest that delight should be lost forever.

In the transcendent state desire and dread are ended; and the thirst for gain and the fear of loss are things that are no more; for where the universal order is seen, universal good is seen; and where perennial joy in that good is a normal condition, what is there left to desire, what remains to be feared?

He who has brought his entire nature into conformity and harmony with the law of righteousness, who has made his thoughts pure, and his deeds blameless, he it is who has entered into liberty. He has transcended darkness and mortality, and has passed into light and immortality. For the transcendent state is at first a higher order of morality, then a new form of perception, and at last a comprehensive understanding of the universal moral causation. And this morality, this vision, and this understanding constitute the new consciousness, the divine life.

The transcendent man is he who is above and beyond the dominion of self; he has transcended evil, and lives in the practice and knowledge of good. He is like a man who, having long looked upon the world with darkened eyes, is now restored to sight, and sees things as they are.

Evil is an experience, and not a power. If it were an independent power in the universe, it could not be transcended by any being. But though not real as a power, it is real as a condition, an experience, for all experience is of the nature of reality. It is a state of ignorance of undevelopment, and as such it recedes and disappears before the light of knowledge, as the intellectual ignorance of the child vanishes before the gradually accumulating learning, or as darkness dissolves before the rising light.

The painful experiences of evil pass away as the new experiences of good enter into and possess the field of consciousness. And what are the new experiences of good? They are many and beautiful — such as the joyful knowledge of freedom from sin; the absence of remorse; deliverance from all the torments of temptation; ineffable joy in conditions and circumstances which formerly caused deep affliction; imperviousness to hurt by the actions of others; great patience and sweetness of character; serenity of mind under all circumstances; emancipation from doubt, fear, and anxiety; freedom from all dislike, envy, and enmity, with the power to feel and act kindly towards those who see fit to constitute themselves one's enemies or opponents; the divine power to give blessings for curses, and to return good for evil; a deep knowledge of the human heart, with a perception of its fundamental goodness; insight into the law of moral causation and the mental evolution of beings, with a prophetic foresight of the sublime good that awaits humanity; and above all, a glad rejoicing in the limitation and impotency of evil, and in the eternal supremacy and power of good. All these, and the calm, strong, far-reaching life that these imply and contain, are the rich experiences of the transcendent man, along with all the new and varied resources, the vast powers, the quickened abilities, and enlarged capacities that spring to life in the new consciousness.

Transcendence is transcendent virtue. Evil and good cannot dwell together. Evil must be abandoned, left behind and transcended, before good is grasped and known, and when good is practised and fully comprehended, then all the afflictions of the mind are at an end, for that which is accompanied with pain and sorrow in the consciousness of evil is not so accompanied in the consciousness of good. Whatsoever happens to the good man cannot cause him perplexity or sorrow, for he knows its cause and issue, knows the good which it is ordained to accomplish in himself, and so his mind remains happy and serene. Though the body of the good man be bound, his mind is free; though it be wounded and in pain, joy and peace abide within his heart.

A spiritual teacher had a pupil who was apt and earnest. After several years of learning and practice the pupil one day propounded a question which his master could not answer. After days of deep meditation, the master said to his pupil: "I cannot answer the question which you have asked; have you any solution to offer?" Whereupon the pupil formulated a reply to the question which he had propounded; and the master said to him: "You have answered that which I could not, and henceforth nor I nor any man can instruct you, for now you are indeed instructed by truth. You have soared, like the kingly eagle, where no man can follow. Your work is now to instruct others. You are no longer the pupil, you have become the master."

In looking back on the self-life which he has transcended, the divinely enlightened man sees that all the afflictions of that life were his schoolmasters teaching him, and leading him upward, and that in the measure that he penetrated their meaning, and lifted himself above them, they departed from him. Their mission to teach him having ended, they left him triumphant master of the field; for the lower cannot teach the higher; ignorance cannot instruct wisdom; evil cannot enlighten good; nor can the pupil set lessons for the master. That which is transcended cannot reach up to that which transcends. Evil can only teach in its own sphere, where it is regarded as a master; in the sphere of good it has no place, no authority.

The strong traveller on the highroad of truth knows no such thing as resignation to evil; he knows only obedience to good. He who submits to evil, saying, "Sin cannot be overcome, and evil must be borne," thereby acknowledges that evil is his master; and not his master to instruct him, but to bind and oppress him. The lover of good cannot also be a lover of evil, nor can he, for one moment, admit its ascendency. He elevates and glorifies good, not evil. He loves light, not darkness. When a man makes truth his master, he abandons error; and as he transcends error, he becomes more like his master, until at last he becomes one with truth, teaching it, as a master, by his actions, and reflecting it in his life.

Transcendence is not an abnormal condition; it belongs to the orderly process of evolution; and though, as yet, few have reached it, all will come into it in the course of the ages. And he who ascends into it, sins no more, sorrows no more, and is no more troubled; good are his thoughts, good are his actions, and good is the tranquil tenor of his way. He has conquered self, and has submitted to truth; he has mastered evil, and has comprehended good. Hence-forth nor men nor books can instruct him, for he is instructed by the Supreme Good, even the spirit of truth.

BEATITUDE

When divine good is practised, life is bliss. Bliss is the normal condition of the good man; and those outer assaults, harassments, and persecutions which bring such sufferings to others, only serve to heighten his happiness, for they cause the deep fountain of good within him to well up in greater abundance.

To have transcendent virtue is to enjoy transcendent felicity. The beatific blessedness which Jesus holds out is promised to those having the beatific virtues — to the merciful, the pure in heart, the peacemakers, and so on. The higher virtue does not merely and only lead to happiness, it is happiness. It is impossible for a man of transcendent virtue to be unhappy. The cause of unhappiness must be sought and found in the self-loving elements, and not in the self-sacrificing qualities. A man may have virtue, and be unhappy, but not so if he have divine virtue. Human virtue is mingled with self, and therefore with sorrow; but from divine virtue every taint of self has been purged away, and with it every vestige of misery. One comparison will suffice to illustrate this: a man may have the courage of a lion in attack and self-defence (such courage being a human virtue), but he will not thereby be rendered supremely happy; but he whose courage is of that divine kind which enables him to transcend both attack and defence, and to remain mild, serene, and lovable under attack, such a man will thereby be rendered supremely happy. Moreover, his assailant will be rendered more happy, in that his more powerful good will overcome and cast out the fierce and unhappy evil of the other.

The acquisition of human virtue is a great step towards truth; but the divine way transcends it, — truth lies upward and beyond.

Doing good in order to gain a personal heaven or personal Immortality is human virtue, but it is not unmixed with self, and not emancipated from sorrow. In the transcendent virtues all is good, and good is all, and there is no personal or ulterior aim. Human virtue is imperfect; it is mixed with the baser, selfish elements, and needs to be transmuted. Divine virtue is unblemished, pure; it is complete and perfect in itself.

And what are the transcendent virtues that embody all felicity? They are:

Impartiality; the seeing so deeply into the human heart, and into human actions, that it becomes impossible to take sides with one man or one party against another, and therefore the power to be perfectly just.

Unlimited Kindness towards all men and all creatures, whether enemies or friends.

Perfect Patience at all times, in all circumstances, and under the severest trials.

Profound Humility; the total abnegation of self; the judging of one's own actions as though they were the actions of another.

Stainless Purity of mind and deed. Freedom from all evil thoughts and impure imaginings.

Unbroken Calmness of mind, even in the midst of outward strife, or surrounded by the turmoil of many vicissitudes.

Abiding Goodness of heart; imperviousness to evil; returning good for evil.

Compassion; deep pity for all creatures and beings in their sufferings. Shielding the weak and helpless; and protecting, out of pity, even one's enemies from injury and slander.

Abounding Love toward all living things; rejoicing with the happy and successful, and sympathizing with the sorrowing and defeated.

Perfect Peace toward all things. Being at peace with all the world. A profound reconciliation to the Divine Order of the universe.

Such are the virtues that transcend both vice and virtue. They include all that virtue embodies, while going beyond it into divine truth. They are the fruits of innumerable efforts to achieve; the glorious gifts of him that overcomes; they constitute the ten-jewelled crown prepared for the calm brow of him who has conquered himself. With these majestic virtues is the mind of the sage adorned. By them he is eternally shielded from sin and sorrow, from harm and hurt, from trouble and turmoil. In them he abides in a happiness, a blessedness, a bliss, so pure and tranquil, so deep and high, so far transcending all the fleeting excitements of self, as to be unknown and incomprehensible to the self-seeking consciousness.

The sage has conquered passion, and has come to lasting peace. As the mighty mountain remains unmoved by the turbulent ocean that beats round its base, so the mind of the sage, towering in lofty virtue, remains unshaken by the tempests of passion which beat unceasingly upon the shores of life.

Good and wise, he is evermore happy and serene; transcendently virtuous, he lives in beatific bliss.

PEACE

Where passion is, peace is not; where peace is, passion is not. To know this is to master the first letter in the divine language of perfect deeds; for to know that passion and peace cannot dwell together is to be well prepared to renounce the lesser and embrace the greater.

Men pray for peace, yet cling to passion; they foster strife, yet pray for heavenly rest. This is ignorance, profound spiritual ignorance; it is not to know the first letter in the alphabet of things divine.

Hatred and love, strife and peace, cannot dwell together in the same heart. Where one is admitted as a welcome guest, the other will be turned away as an unwelcome stranger. He who despises another will be despised by others; he who opposes his fellow-man will himself be resisted. He should not be surprised, and mourn, that men are divided. He should know that he is propagating strife. He should understand his lack of peace.

He is brave who conquers another; but he who conquers himself is supremely noble. He who is victorious over another may in turn be defeated; but he who overcomes himself will never be subdued.

By the way of self-conquest is the Perfect Peace achieved. Man cannot understand it, cannot approach it, until he sees the supreme necessity of turning away from the fierce fighting of things without, and entering upon the noble warfare against evils within. He is already on the Saintly Way who has realized that the enemy of the world is within, and not without; that his own ungoverned thoughts are the source of confusion and strife; that his own unchastened desires are the violaters of his peace, and of the peace of the world.

If a man has conquered lust and anger, hatred and pride, selfishness and greed, he has conquered the world; he has slain the enemies of peace, and peace remains with him.

Peace does not fight; is not a partisan; has no blatant voice. The triumph of peace is an unassailable silence.

He who is overcome by force is not thereby overcome in his heart; he may be a greater enemy than before; but he who is overcome by the spirit of peace is thereby changed at heart. He that was an enemy has become a friend. Force and strife work upon the passions and fears, but love and peace reach and reform the heart.

The pure-hearted and wise have peace in their hearts; it enters into their actions; they apply it in their lives. It is more powerful than strife; it conquers where force would fail. Its wings shield the righteous. Under its protection, the harmless are not harmed. It affords a secure shelter from the heat of selfish struggle. It is a refuge for the defeated, a tent for the lost, and a temple for the pure.

When peace is practised, and possessed, and known, then sin and remorse, grasping and disappointment, craving and temptation, desiring and grieving — all the turbulence and torment of the mind — are left behind in the dark sphere of self to which they belong, and beyond which they cannot go. Beyond where these dark spectres move, bask in Eternal Light the radiant Plains of Divine Beatitude, and to these the traveller on the High and Holy Way comes in due time. From the binding swamps of passion, through the thorny forests of many vanities, across the arid deserts of doubt and despair, he travels on, not turning back, nor staying his course, but ever moving toward his sublime destination, until at last he comes, a meek and lowly yet strong and radiant conqueror, to the Beautiful City of Peace.

JAMES ALLEN QUOTES

"No duty is more urgent than that of returning thanks."

"The man who does not shrink from self-crucifixion can never fail to accomplish the object upon which the heart is set."

"You are today where your thoughts have brought you."

"In all human affairs there are efforts, and there are results, and the strength of the effort is the measure of the result."

"Men are anxious to improve their circumstances but are unwilling to improve themselves; they therefore remain bound."

"A man is literally what he thinks."

"A man has to learn that he cannot command things but that he can command himself; that he cannot coerce the wills of others but that he can mold and master his own will; and things serve him who serves Truth; people seek guidance of him who is master of himself."

"You will become as small as your controlling desire; as great as your dominant aspiration."

"As you think, you travel, and as you love, you attract."

"Self-control is strength."

"Right thought is mastery."

"The more tranquil a man becomes, the greater is his success, his influence, his power for good. Calmness of mind is one of the beautiful jewels of wisdom."

"Not what he wishes and prays for does a man get but what he justly earns. His wishes and prayers are only gratified and answered when they harmonize with his thoughts and actions."

"Man is made or unmade by himself. By the right choice he ascends. As a being of power, intelligence, and love, and the commander of his own thoughts, he holds the key to every situation."

"Calmness is power."

"Cherish your visions. Cherish your ideals. Cherish the music that stirs in your heart, the beauty that forms in your mind, the loveliness that drapes your purest thoughts. For out of them will grow all delightful conditions, all heavenly environment, of these, if you but remain true to him, your world will at last be built."

"You will never do anything in this world without courage. It is the greatest quality of the mind next to honor."

"They who have conquered doubt and fear have conquered failure."

"A man only begins to be a man when he ceases to whine and revile. And builds himself up in strong and noble thoughts; ceases to kick against circumstances but begins to use them as aids to his more rapid progress, and as a means of the hidden powers and possibilities within himself."

"Let your soul expand, let your heart reach out to others in loving and generous warmth, and great and lasting will be your joy, and all prosperity will come to you."

"The dreamers are the saviors of the worlds."

"Dream lofty dreams, and as you dream, so you shall become, your vision is the promise of what you shall one day be; your ideal is the prophecy of what you shall at last unveil."

"The outer conditions of a person's life will always be found to reflect their inner beliefs."

"A person is only by the thoughts that he chooses."

"Circumstances do not make the man, they reveal him."

"The law of harvest is to reap more than you sow. Sow an act, and you reap a habit. Sow a habit and you reap a character. Sow a character and you reap a destiny."

"Harmony is one phase of the law whose spiritual expression is love."

"Work joyfully and peacefully, knowing that right thoughts and right efforts inevitably bring about right results."

"A man sooner or later discovers that he is the master-gardener of his soul, the director of his life."

"As a man thinketh in his heart, so shall he be."

"Our life is what our thoughts make it. A man will find that as he alters his thoughts toward things and other people, things and other people will alter towards him."

"It is a process of diverting one's scattered forces into one powerful channel."

"Men do not attract which they want but that which they are."

"He who would accomplish little must sacrifice little; he who would accomplish much must sacrifice much."

"All that a man achieves and all that he fails to achieve is the direct result of his own thoughts."

"A man becomes calm in the measure that he understands himself as a thought-evolved being. For such knowledge necessitates the understanding of others as the result of thought, and as he develops a right understanding, and sees ever more clearly the internal relations of things by the action of cause and effect, he ceases to fuss, fume, worry, and grieve. He remains poised, steadfast, serene."

"The law of harvest is to reap more than you sow. Sow an act, and you reap a habit. Sow a habit and you reap a character. Sow a character and you reap a destiny. "

"There can be no progress nor achievement without sacrifice, and a man's worldly success will be by the measure that he sacrifices his confused animal thoughts, and fixes his mind on the development of his plans, and the strengthening of his resolution and self-reliance."

"Man is made or unmade by himself. By the right choice he ascends. As a being of power, intelligence, and love, and the lord of his own thoughts, he holds the key to every situation..."

"All that a man achieves and all that he fails to achieve is the direct result of his own thoughts."

"The visions you glorify in your mind,
The ideals you enthrone in your heart..
This you will build your life by...
This you will become."

"A noble and God-like character is not a thing of favor or chance, but is the natural result of continued effort in right thinking, the effect of long-cherished association with God-like thoughts."

"A particular train of thought persisted in, be it good or bad, cannot fail to produce its results on the character and circumstances. A man cannot directly choose his circumstances, but he can choose his thoughts, and so indirectly, yet surely, shape his circumstances."

"Good thoughts and actions can never produce bad results; bad thoughts and actions can never produce good results ... We understand this law in the natural world, and work with it; but few understand it in the mental and moral world—although its operation there is just as simple and undeviating— and they, therefore, do not cooperate with it."

"The dreamers are the saviors of the world. As the visible world is sustained by the invisible, so men, through all their trials and sins and sordid vocations, are nourished by the beautiful visions of their solitary dreamers."

"Do not dwell upon the sins and mistakes of yesterday so exclusively as to have no energy and mind left for living rightly today, and do not think that the sins of yesterday can prevent you from living purely today."

"Men are anxious to improve their circumstances, but are unwilling to improve themselves."

"He who would accomplish little need sacrifice little; he who would achieve much must sacrifice much. He who would attain highly must sacrifice greatly."

"You are today where your thoughts have brought you;
you will be tomorrow where your thoughts take you."

"The more tranquil a man becomes, the greater is his success, his influence, his power for good. Calmness of mind is one of the beautiful jewels of wisdom."

"A man only begins to be a man when he ceases to whine and revile, and commences to search for the hidden justice which regulates his life. And he adapts his mind to that regulating factor, he ceases to accuse others as the cause of his condition, and builds himself up in strong and noble thoughts; ceases to kick against circumstances, but begins to use them as aids to his more rapid progress, and as a means of the hidden powers and possibilities within himself."

"A strong man cannot help a weaker unless the weaker is willing to be helped, and even then the weak man must become strong of himself; he must, by his own efforts, develop the strength which he admires in another. None but himself can alter his condition."

"A man's mind may be likened to a garden, which may be intelligently cultivated or allowed to run wild; but whether cultivated or neglected, it must, and will, bring forth. If no useful seeds are put into it, then an abundance of useless weed seeds will fall therein, and will continue to produce their kind."

"The outer conditions of a person's life will always be found to be harmoniously related to his inner state...Men do not attract that which they want, but that which they are."

❑❑❑

9 789388 841399

Printed at Repro India Ltd.